Rescue Acupressure:
Instantly Suppress Stress, Headaches, Memory Lapses In Desperate Situations Like During An Exam.
By Remy Roulier

Disclaimer

TABLE OF CONTENTS

TRIGGER INSTANT RELIEF... WITH THE TOUCH OF YOUR FINGER!

Dear reader,

Thank you for purchasing this book and congratulations!...

...Because this may be the best investment you will ever make for both your health and success.

Here is why:

Each year, 80% of Doctor's visits are due to pain in general, because body or emotional pain can happen at any time and at any moment of your life.

If some people are lucky enough because they managed to prevent pain by an early visit at the doctor, others can see a particular pain suddenly appear in the worst moment of their life.

This is particularly true for students, where anxiety, stress, headaches or memory losses can smartly select the most vicious moment to show up: the moment when students are taking their final exam...

...And thus ruin in a few minutes **a whole year** of hard studying efforts, sometimes until late in the night reading, learning, reading and learning again.

Such a scenario can happen to anyone, especially to students who are generally in good health and thus not prepared to cope with such events that can lead to real disasters.

No one is safe from a violent headache that suddenly appears 27 minutes after the beginning of the GRE, LSAT, GMAT or any other important exam.

The minutes are counting down, and no way for the student to focus again on the exam.

In this case, there will be no doctor, no pills...And no miraculous method to instantly relieve this headache, as if by magic.

Unfortunately for the student, it will almost always result in a grade poor as a church mouse, and an exam brilliantly failed. Worst of all, the $10000 dollars or more of his or her academic year will vanish...like a shadow in the night.

This book will reveal you an amazing method to **never** let this happen to you.

Because at the end of this book, you will have become your own therapist.

You will master an extremely simple and efficient healing technique developed by oriental doctors, with amazing advantages that make it almost unrealistic and magic because...

...You will be able to:

1- Relieve the 11 worst students' pains: anxiety, calm and tranquility, energy, exhaustion, fatigue, headaches, memory losses, nervosity, sleep, stage fright, vitality.

2- Relieve these pains **instantly**.

3- Use the technique **anywhere**.

4- Use the technique **when you want**.

5- Use the technique **discretely**, without anyone noticing.

6- Master the technique **immediately** upon finishing this book.

And best of all, you will be able to do all this:

7- Only with the touch of your finger!

Right now, let's raise the red curtain to discover the amazing technique that will make you become a master in the management of the worst students pains:

It is called...the G-JO.

Part 1:
WHAT IS THE G-JO

1.1- Definition of the G-JO

Acupuncture is today recognized worldwide by the National Institute of Health (NIH) and the World Health Organization (WHO) for its outstanding ability to successfully treat a wide range of disorders naturally.

Researches carried by oriental and world renowned doctors allowed the discovery of an extremely simple and efficient method of manual application of acupuncture, avoiding to use needles that require a specialist.

This technique is called the G-JO, and consists in a fingertip stimulation of specific points on the body.

G-JO is the translation of ideograms meaning "first aid".

The G-JO will guide you and give you the ability to easily and instantly suppress fatigue, stimulate your memory, relieve headaches, stress and...any of the 7 other pains previously described.

And all this absolutely anywhere, without anyone noticing...

...Like in a lecture amphitheater, a study classroom, or **in an examination room**.

1.2- Precautions

You should use the G-JO as an additional help, that is exactly in the primary sense of its meaning: first-aid.

It can't be used as a background therapy. If you suffer from deep fatigue, important memory losses or extremely frequent headaches, you **must** consult a doctor.

You must not use the G-JO in the following cases:

- Treat a chronic or persistent disease.

- Within the 4 hours after the absorption of medication or drugs.

- Within the 30 minutes that immediately follow a big meal, an intense physical effort, a hot bath.

- If you are under medical treatment.

- If you are subject to internal bleeding caused by external stimulation, in the case of purpura, ulcer, hemophilia or aneurysm.

- If you suffer from heart disorder or cellular tissue disease (chronic arthrisis, cancer, cataract, tumor, varicose veins).

- For pregnant women.

- If the G-JO point is under a scar, wart, mole or in an inflamed or swollen region.

The G-JO is attended to healthy people. It only provides temporary relief.

A symptom is often the sign of an underlying medical problem; if the symptom you try to treat subsists, consult your doctor.

***

Finally, an excessive stimulation of the indicated points may become harmful. Stimulating 10 times per day the points that correspond to memory won't increase your memory by 10. It's possible to stimulate 2 to 4 times per day the same points during 2 to 3 days according to your needs, but it should not last longer.

***

Part 2:
HOW TO PROCEED

You can proceed with these 2 simple steps:

Step 1:

Locate the exact pressure point corresponding to the effect you expect.

Step 2:

Stimulate the pressure point.

2.1- How to Locate with Accuracy the G-JO Point

Each location can vary slightly from one person to another.

The measurement units to locate the G-JO points are the hand width and the thumb width according to the pictures below:

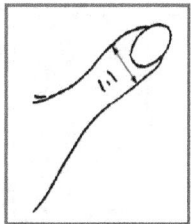 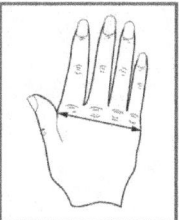

For instance, the point N°77 is located on the inner edge of the arm, at one hand width and two thumb widths under the flexion crease of the wrist (in direction of the elbow) in the axis of the pinkie, according to the picture hereafter:

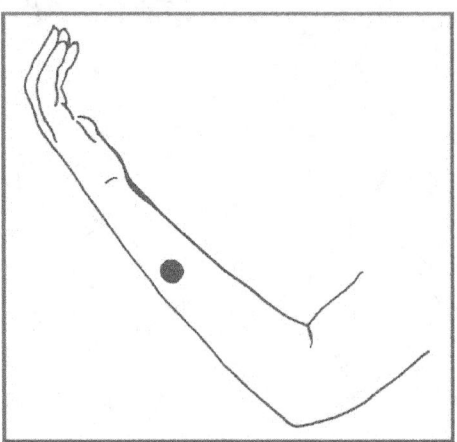

To find it, place your hand under the flexion crease of the wrist, locate mentally the line that delimits your hand, place the edge of your thumb on this line, locate mentally the line that delimits your thumb and then place the edge of your thumb on this line.

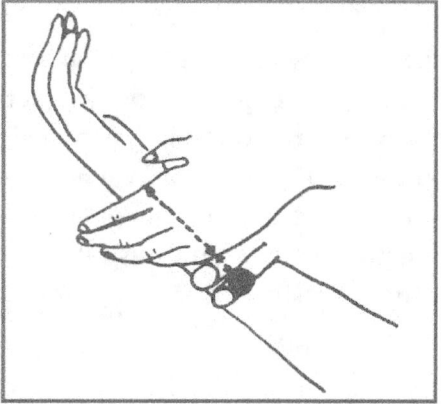

Most of the G-JO points have their symmetrical point on the other half of the body.

Thus, the point N°77 in this example is located on the right arm and also on the left arm. <u>You will always have to stimulate the 2 points</u>.

If you want to use the G-JO on someone else, you will have to use <u>his or her</u> thumb and <u>his or her</u> hand as measurement units on <u>his or her</u> body.

The points' location may vary slightly from one person to another. So, the indicated position on the pictures corresponds more to a region than a precise location. To accurately find the G-JO point, you will want to explore the indicated region until you start feeling a kind of twinge, a particularly sensitive place. Don't hesitate to exert a strong pressure with the fingertip.

2.2- How to Stimulate a G-JO Point

Massage the G-JO point clockwise. Massage it quickly and in <u>depth</u> with the fingertip by exerting a strong pressure (about 22 lbs).

This stimulation should last 15 to 20 seconds.

<u>Immediately after</u>, repeat the same operation on the symmetrical point.

Don't do a stimulation with long nails. You can use the tip of a pencil (not sharp) or the joint of your finger.

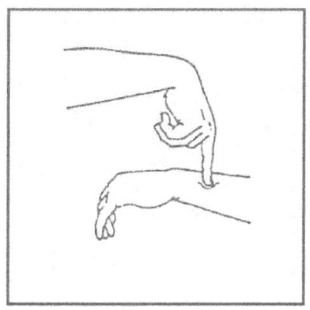 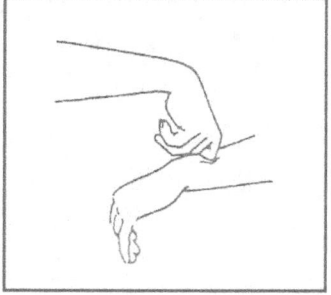

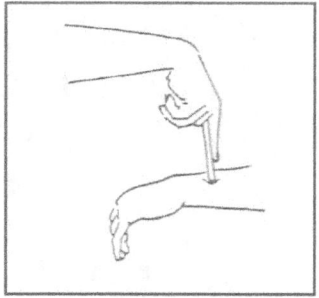

The pressure on the point must be strong but <u>shouldn't cause</u> a bruise.

It's recommended to relax a few moments before starting the stimulation of the G-JO points.

Don't forget that each point has its symmetrical exactly at the same place on the other half of the body. You always have to stimulate the 2 points one after the other.

You can start indifferently from the right or the left point.

Part 3:
PRACTICAL APPLICATIONS

The application range of the G-JO is really wide, it can relieve a large amount of troubles or diseases, but in this case it has to be exclusively performed by a specialist.

As said previously, this book is specially focused on what is useful for students in their daily life, that is:

Anxiety - Calm & Tranquility - Energy - Exhaustion - Fatigue - Headaches - Memory - Nervosity - Sleep - Stage Fright - Vitality.

*** Attention ***

FOR ANY OF THESE APPLICATIONS, SEVERAL G-JO POINTS ARE INDICATED. AS SOON AS THE STIMULATION OF ONE OF THEM PRODUCES THE EFFECT YOU WANT, IT IS ABSOLUTELY USELESS TO STIMULATE THE OTHER POINTS.

***

3.1- Anxiety

Definition:

Justified or unjustified apprehension of an upcoming event or situation. This generally translates into a difficulty to breathe with a sensation of weight or of knot in the pit of the stomach, and may be accompanied by pale face and cooling of the body extremities.

Points to Stimulate:

15 (especially in case of stage fright), 69, 71.

3.2- Calm & Tranquility

Definition:
(Also see anxiety and nervosity). Points to use in case of minor nervosity with no link with serious problems.

Points to Stimulate:
13, 17.

3.3- Energy

Definition:

Any deficiency or excess requires a change in diet, lifestyle, activity and/or treatment.

A slight stimulation will bring you a temporary energy boost. A quick stimulation will allow you to reduce your energy overflow.

Points to Stimulate:

<u>6</u>, <u>9</u>, <u>69</u>, <u>97</u>.

3.4- Exhaustion

Definition:

(See fatigue). Exhaustion is caused by extended or too important physical or mental efforts. It is generally characterized by a total apathy, a great weakness, dizziness, etc.

Points to Stimulate:

21, 38, 97.

3.5- Fatigue

Definition:

(See energy, exhaustion, vitality). Less severe than exhaustion, it manifests itself through an important loss of vitality, of dynamism and through a more or less important weariness. It's the result of an excess of physical or intellectual work. Fatigue impairs the faculties of sensorial perception, attention and memory.

Fatigue has to be treated <u>as soon as it appears</u> in order to avoid an accumulation that could become very harmful.

Points to Stimulate:

<u>9</u>, <u>21</u>, <u>97</u>.

3.6- Headaches

Definition:

They can be the result of multiple problems and diseases. If they persist, consult your doctor. Among students, they can also be caused by untreated poor eyesight or bad reading lighting.

Points to Stimulate:

1, 4, 9, 10, 13, (and 15 if the pain is due to anxiety), 38, 64, 68, (and 69, if pain in the top of the skull).

3.7- Memory

Definition:

Memory troubles can be caused by intellectual fatigue and/or by various problems (anxiety, apprehension, nutritional deficiency, use of various drugs, etc.).

Any sudden memory loss can hide a serious problem, consult a doctor as soon as possible.

Points to Stimulate:

1, 10, 78.

3.8- Nervosity

Definition:

It is characterized by an impulsive and irrational behavior, an useless over-activity, a lack of mental balance and calmness.

Points to Stimulate:

13, 17. And also, massage the hands especially around the wrists.

3.9- Sleep

Definition:

A need of sleep can be simply due to tiredness, in this case rest is the best treatment.

On the contrary, an excessive need of sleep is often a symptom of a psychological problem and/or of an inappropriate diet.

Points to Stimulate:
64, 68, 97.

3.10- Stage Fright

(See anxiety, nervosity.)

3.11- Vitality

Definition:

(See energy). It represents the natural expression of life, the aggressive energy (taken here in the sense of moving forward), the determination, the resistance and the power of will.

Points to Stimulate:

65, 108.

Remember that it's useless to stimulate all the points indicated to obtain the desired result.
Stimulate the first point indicated as well as the symmetrical point: if you obtain the desired effect, stop, don't stimulate the other points.

Part 4:
ILLUSTRATION OF THE
G-JO POINTS

Point N°1

Headaches. Memory.

Starting from the crease of the wrist, the point is located at 1.5 thumb width above.

You can use the picture below to find it: the point is located under the extremity of your forefinger, in a small hollow.

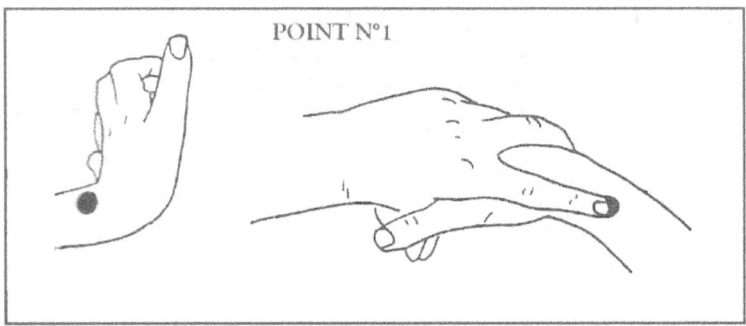

POINT N°1

Point N°4

Headaches.

Starting from the crease of the wrist, the point is located on the back of the forearm at 2 thumb widths above, in line with the middle finger.

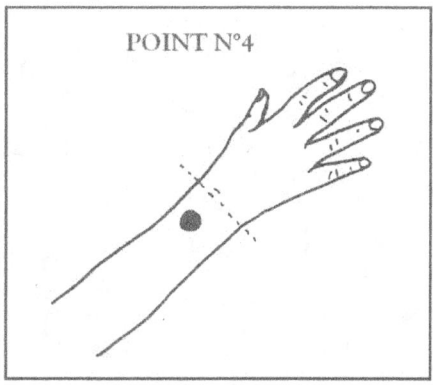

Point N°6

Energy.

In the vertical axis of the navel at one hand width under it.

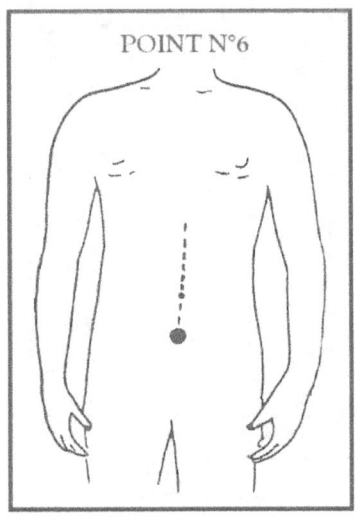

Point N°9

Energy. Fatigue. Headaches.

In the patella-ankle axis, at one hand width under the patella, then at one thumb width towards the outside of the leg. In the hole formed by the shin.

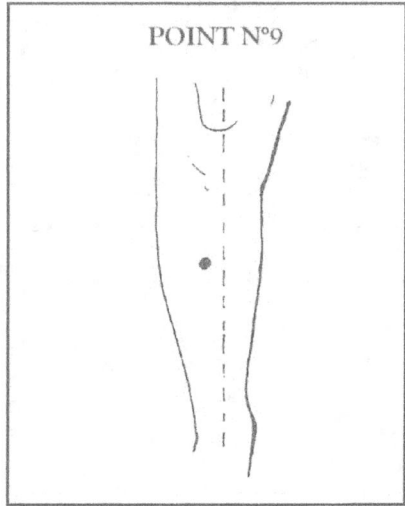

POINT N°9

Point N°10

Headaches. Memory.

On the inside of the forearm, in line with the middle finger, at 2 thumb widths above the crease of the wrist.

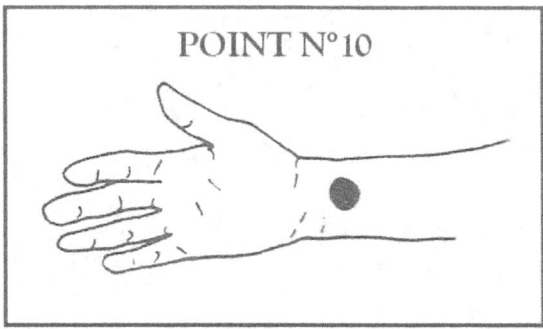

Point N°13

**Headaches. Calm & Tranquility.
Nervosity (in this last case, stimulate also the point n°17)**

Tighten the thumb and the forefinger, place your finger at the top of the bulge of flesh, relax the hand while keeping your finger on the point indicated.

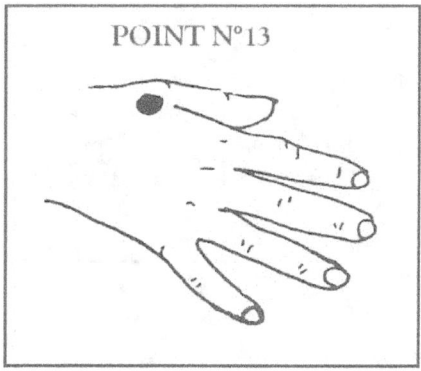

POINT N°13

Point N°15

Anxiety. Headaches.

On the internal side of the wrist, in line with the pinkie, in the crease of the wrist.

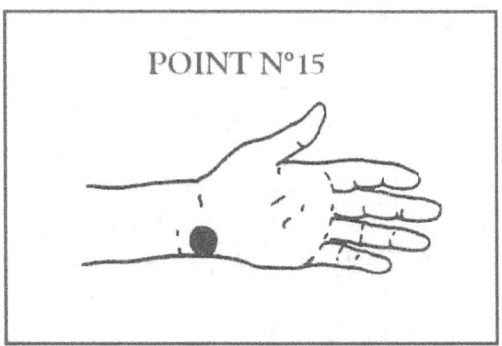

Point N°17

Calm & Tranquility. Nervosity.

On the foot, in the separation axis between the big toe and
the second toe, at 2 thumb widths above.

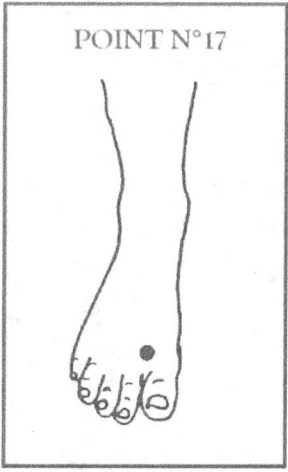

Point N°21

Exhaustion and physical fatigue.

On the top of the shoulders. Raise the arm a little bit above the level of the shoulder and place your finger in the hollow thus formed, the one which is located furthest forward. Keep your finger in this hollow, lower the arm and start the stimulation.

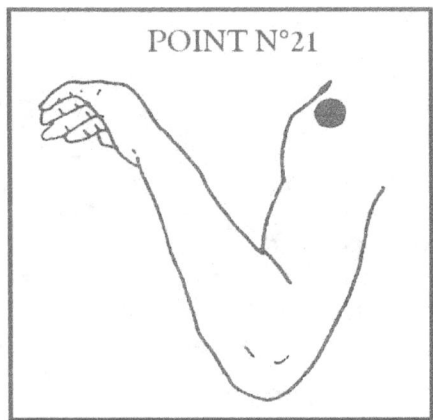

POINT N°21

Point N°38

Headaches. Physical exhaustion.

On the back of the hand, on the separation line between the ring finger and the pinkie, at 1.5 thumb width above.

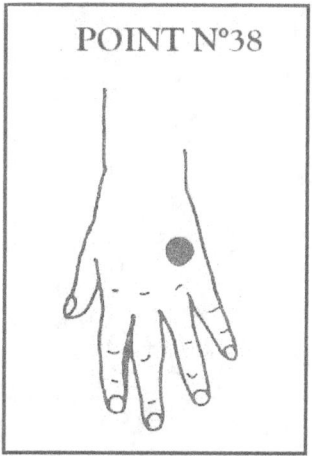

Point N°64

Headaches. Sleep.

On the 4th toe, immediately after the nail, slightly outwards.

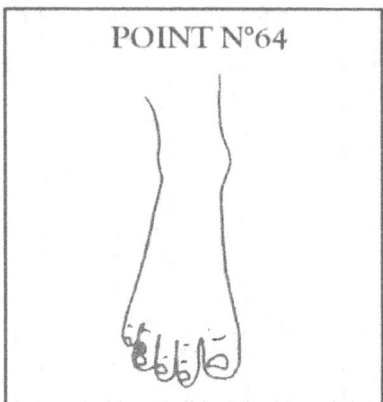

Point N°65

Vitality.

On the outer edge of the leg, at 2 hand widths above the top of the ankle bone and slightly behind a vertical axis that would start from the ankle.

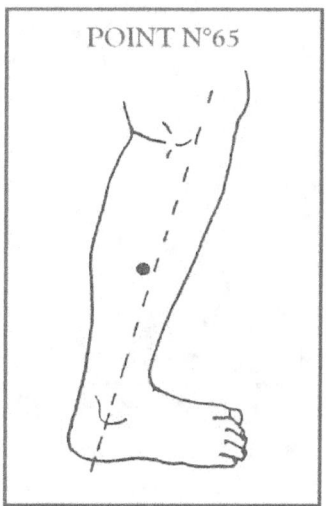

Point N°68

Sleep. Headaches.

On the big toe, just above the inner corner of the nail.

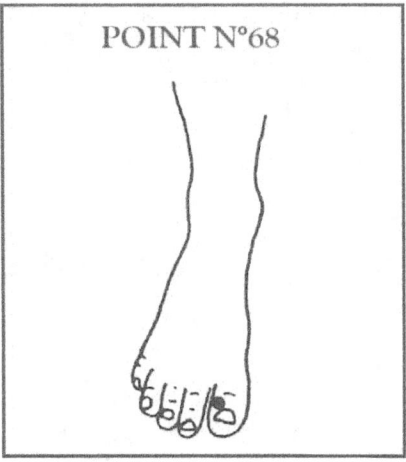

Point N°69

Anxiety. Headaches. Energy.

On the sole of the foot, at the center of the beginning of the foot arch.

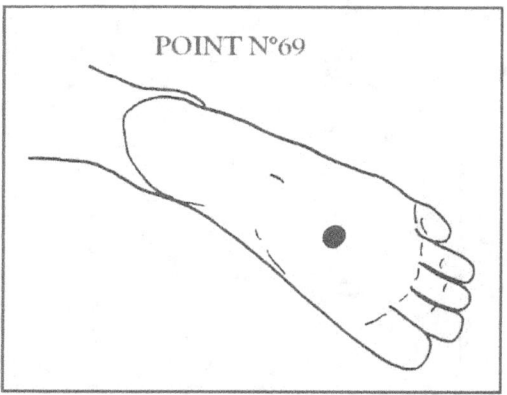

Point N°71

Anxiety.

On the internal side of the foot. On an axis starting from the top of the ankle bone and that extends to the extremity of the tail, at 2 thumb widths from the extremity of the tail.

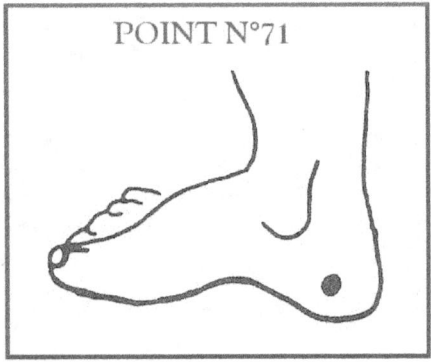

Point N°78

Memory.

On the external side of the arm, at 2 hand widths below the top of the shoulder.

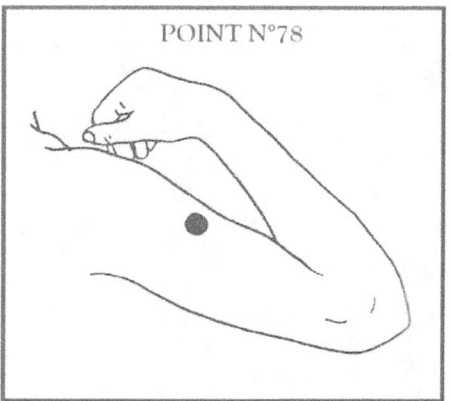

Point N°97

Fatigue. Energy. Exhaustion. Sleep.

At the same level of the nipples, at the center of sternum.
For women, it's better to measure from the base of the
neck, at 2 hand widths below.

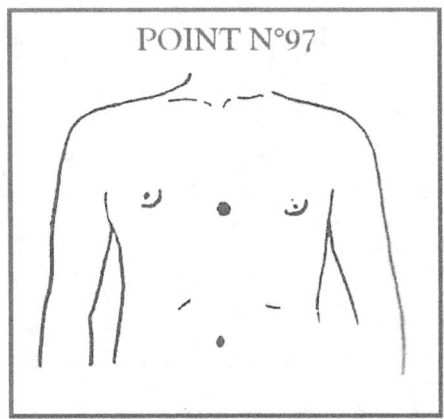

Point N°108

Vitality.

Behind the head at one hand width above the base of the skull in the axis of the top of the ears.

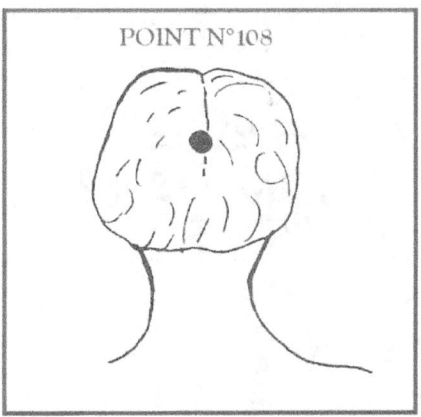

Part 5:
SUMMARY

What to Remember:

- RESPECT THE PRECAUTIONS FOR USE.

- LOCATE THE G-JO POINT THAT CORRESPONDS TO THE DESIRED EFFECT.

- STIMULATE THE G-JO POINT BY MASSAGING IT CLOCKWISE.

- MASSAGE QUICKLY AND IN DEPTH.

- REPEAT THE SAME OPERATION <u>IMMEDIATELY AFTER</u> ON THE SYMMETRICAL POINT.

- SEVERAL G-JO POINTS ARE INDICATED FOR A SAME APPLICATION. AS SOON AS THE STIMULATION OF ONE OF THEM PRODUCES THE DESIRED EFFECT, IT IS USELESS TO STIMULATE THE OTHERS.

- REMEMBER BY HEART THE LOCATION OF THE POINT CORRESPONDING TO HEADACHES, MEMORY AND STAGE FRIGHT, YOU MAY NEED THEM DURING YOUR EXAM.

CONGRATULATIONS

The final thought of this book is specially addressed to you and holds in one word:

CONGRATULATIONS!...

...Because you have finished this book, which means that starting from now, you are able to instantly relieve any of the worst students pains anywhere and when you want, for you and also for the others...only with the touch of your finger!

All you have to do is to let the secrets of this book guide you.

They will give you a real advantage over 99% of people or more, because there's a lot to bet that they have never heard of this amazing technique, contrary to you.

Keep this book preciously, because it will be extremely helpful not only for your exams but also in your daily life, forever.

I wish you the best success in your exams and in your life, from the bottom of my heart.

MORE BOOKS FROM THE AUTHOR

HOW TO CONCENTRATE LIKE EINSTEIN:
THE LAZY STUDENT'S WAY TO INSTANTLY IMPROVE MEMORY & GRADES WITH THE DOCTOR VITTOZ SECRET CONCENTRATION TECHNIQUE

Concentrate now on what you want as long as you want by learning the never before revealed concentration technique used by Einstein.

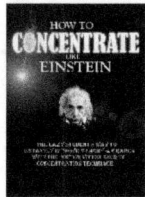

DETOX DIET:
EATING WELL FOR A LIFE OF PURE ENERGY, SHAPE AND HEALTH

All you need to know about eating well to get an exceptional health and shape is inside this book. Discover now the true principles to eating well (4 powers and 4 poisons) that will completely detoxify you and allow you to create an exceptional health, shape, and energy.

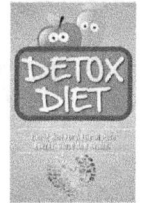

You can also find dozens of other books in French from the author on Amazon.